John Cross Publications

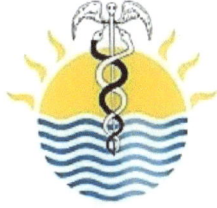

I0116362

Distance Analysis and Healing with the Chakra Energy System – My Way!

John R. Cross FCSP; Dr.Ac.

Chapter Headings

INTRODUCTION

CHAPTER ONE – What is Healing? What is Distant Healing? The Aura. The Major Chakras.

CHAPTER TWO – Dowsing. Dowsing from a list. Making an Analysis Chart

CHAPTER THREE- Analysis of the Major Chakras at the Physical, Etheric, Emotional and Mental levels

CHAPTER FOUR- Distance Healing at the Etheric, Emotional and Mental levels

BIBLIOGRAPHY

INTRODUCTION

This topic is steeped in mystery and intrigue. How can you possibly influence and create changes within the human frame of another person without actually touching them or by not even being in the same room? Distance healing is relatively easy to do (and everyone has the capability to do it) but learning this craft takes time and patience. It is also an emotive topic and easily accepted by some whilst condemned by others who think that anything that is not scientifically proven cannot possibly work.

I have been practising this form of analysis and healing for more years than I care to think of and I would consider myself to be sane, level headed, sensible and all round good egg – far removed from the zany, head-in-the-clouds person that Joe Public would imagine someone who does this to be. I have previously written extensively on the subject of the chakra energy system as well as other 'hands on' therapies so this publication was a natural progression for me in explaining this wonderful form of healing to others. It is the ninth book of mine to be published and is based upon my own research, trial and tribulations and know how. The information in this book is given freely with love and is dedicated to all the long suffering delegates who have studied this method with me and persuaded me to put pen to paper.

As you read through this work you will soon find that all you need to be a successful healer at a distance is to exhibit bags of empathy and love towards your fellow human beings and to able to concentrate with focus and intention to the job in hand. I have purposely used the word 'client' throughout this book and not 'patient', even though as an orthodox medical practitioner for forty years, that is the word I used. However, this topic falls way out of the bounds of conventional medicine.

CHAPTER ONE

What is Distance Analysis? What is Healing? What is Distance Healing? The Aura. The Major Chakras

What is Distance Analysis?

Distance (or distant) analysis is the ability to ascertain information about someone not present. It is generally done by dowsing using a pendulum – the medical word for this being radiesthesia. It is vital that something 'of the client' is used on which to dowse – this may be a blood spot, some hair, a recent photograph or even a signature. These are called 'Witnesses'. [This word is given an upper case initial letter so it isn't confused with a witness of any other kind]. It is even possible that just by writing the client's name down could be sufficient – however this is only to be undertaken by experienced practitioners. The ideal 'Witness' is a small lock of hair in a plastic bag that may be placed on the correct part of the analysis chart. As stated in the Introduction, the requisites for performing distance analysis are two fold – namely to have empathy and love towards your fellow humans (or animals) and to be able to totally concentrate on the job in hand. It is not something to be entertained lightly and financial reward should never ever be the reason for doing it! Each person possesses a unique energy vibration that is often referred to as the PGR (personal general rate). It is this vibration that the practitioner tunes into through the Witness.

What is Healing?

The word 'heal' simply means 'to make whole'. It therefore doesn't necessarily mean 'to cure'. Healing, of course, has many different guises. Each one, though, has a common denominator in that it is the client who heals him/herself with their own complex subtle energy system. All the 'healer' does is to provide the correct stimulus, medicine, treatment, caring, positive words etc. to allow healing to occur. I believe that everyone is capable of healing, be it contact, non-contact or at a distance. There are, though, those amongst us who seem to have a natural gift of healing. This gift is readily accepted by some or denied for many years by others, but eventually driven to it by the still small voice that whispers constantly. Others, including myself, have to 'work at it' over a period of time as practice eventually should make perfect. The many aspects to healing may be categorized as either non-contact or contact healing. Examples of non-contact healing are counselling, hypnotherapy, psychotherapy, radionics, Feng Shui, sound therapy, colour healing and a host of others that may include the giving of homoeopathy, herbs or even allopathic drugs – and never underestimate the power of the placebo effect. Examples of contact healing may include reflexology, osteopathy, chiropractic, shiatsu, physiotherapy, acupuncture and acupressure. These are all forms of healing even though they may not be perceived as such by individual therapists. With each and every type there is an attempt to make the client whole in either mind or body.

What is Distance Healing?

Distance healing is the ability to send healing 'over the ether' via the Witness to the recipient. He or she may be in the next room, next town, next county, or even on the other side of the world. The Witness possesses the total vibrational energy footprint of the individual so any type of thoughts sent through the Witness will be received by the client. I believe that this is possible through what is called the universal or cosmic energy field, simply called 'the field'. It may also be called the collective consciousness.

The Aura

It is impossible to understand and subsequently practice distance healing without accepting that all living matter has an aura. It is fundamental to everything. The knowledge of auras is based upon many traditional views dating back over five thousand years. It is generally understood that there are seven energetic bodies, including the physical body that make up our aura or our energy field emanation. They are Physical, Etheric, Emotional, Mental, Intuitional, Monadic and Divine. Different cultures and philosophies have given these slightly different names. Some very gifted people are able to see auras up to quite a high level. Most people though, with some simple training, are able to see both aspects of the Etheric body up to approximately ten centimetres (four inches) from the skin. My book 'Healing with the Chakra Energy System' –North Atlantic Books (2006) explains the auras in great detail. The knowledge of the auras is essential when using non-contact healing on a client and this knowledge is also used in distance healing with a few refinements. Figure 1.1 below is an illustration showing my interpretation of the aura with the major chakras up to the level of the Mental body– dimensions are given in inches.

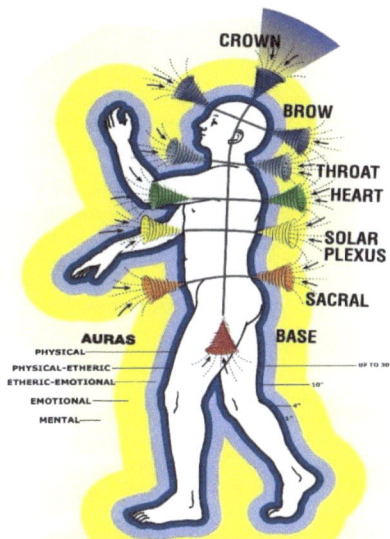

Figure 1.1 The Aura and Major Chakras taken from 'Healing with the Chakra Energy System' poster

It is taken from my best selling A1 colour poster 'Healing with the Chakra Energy System'. The Etheric body is approximately 10 cms or 4" from the skin and is sub divided into the Physical-Etheric at 1" limit and the Etheric-Emotional at 4". The outer limit of the Emotional body is 25cms or 10" and Mental body is 75cms or 30". I have attempted to show in this illustration that the auric bodies become subtler the further away from the physical body. Space only permits illustrating up to the Mental body and in practice that is all you will require. If you can imagine the outer region of the Mental body being 30 inches away from the body, you will soon realise that when we stand close to someone, we can literally be in 'their space' as the two subtle bodies mingle. Taking this on further, the Intuitional, Monadic and Divine bodies are huge distances away. Some schools of thought state that the Divine (or Spiritual) bodies of each living organism on the planet are connected through the soup that is the collective consciousness. The Physical, Etheric, Emotional and Mental Bodies will be discussed in detail in the final chapter.

The Seven Major Chakras

As I have written extensively about the many aspects of the seven major chakras in other tomes, I shall present an outline here and then emphasize their importance in distance healing.

Figure 1.1 shows how the seven major chakras emanating from the physical body in a spiral fashion. They are whorls of energetic matter that link the seven auric layers to the physical body. It is generally agreed in complementary medical circles that we are responsible for our own health and that our emotions play an important part in this. Many of our illnesses, which are represented in the physical body as symptoms, are the result of negative emotional responses to the travails of life. These include birth trauma, the shock of an accident/injury, anxiety and depression and coping with long term grief. These represent a fraction of the constant emotional bombardments that we have to endure day on day. The chakras at the Mental and Emotional levels are affected in that they become congested or over active. This in turn affects the Etheric body and finally the Physical body, giving us symptoms of the energy imbalance that we can see or feel. The type of negative emotion is important. Grief, for example, would affect the Throat chakra (giving throat and bowel symptoms), depression would affect the Solar Plexus chakra (giving a myriad of symptoms affecting the liver, stomach and spleen) and heartache/sadness would affect the Heart chakra (giving us circulatory and mid spinal symptoms). It is therefore important to know, when doing distance analysis and healing, which symptoms of the client are affecting which chakra, because it is the chakra that you the practitioner will help balance in order for the client's symptoms to be alleviated. Some symptoms such as musculo-skeletal conditions are solely within the Physical body, some that include imbalance of our various fluid system you will affect through the Etheric body, some that highlight physical symptoms due to emotional trauma will be affected through the Emotional body and the highest form of distance healing will be through the Mental body. These will be discussed in detail at the end of the chapter on distance healing. Table 1.1 below is a guide showing the various relationships of the major chakras and the presenting symptoms in the physical and emotional bodies that occur with chakra imbalance. It will be shown again (with variations) in the chapter on healing.

	Base	Sacral	Solar Plexus	Heart	Throat	Brow	Crown
NEGATIVE QUALITIES	INSECURITY DOUBT PHOBIAS FEAR NOT GROUNDED ANXIETY FINANCE WORRIES DWELLS ON MATERIALISM OVERWEIGHT TENDENCIES	JEALOUSY ENVY LUST LOW SELF WORTH NYMPHOMANIA OVERWEIGHT TENDENCIES TATS	DEPRESSION WORRY ANXIETY LOW SELF ESTEEM TOO MUCH EMPATHY	TEARFULNESS ANXIETY AFFAIRS OF THE HEART CANNOT FORGIVE OTHERS EXCESS EMPATHY & COMPASSION GIGGLY	SHYNESS INTROVERTNESS PARANOIA POOR EXPRESSION & COMMUNICATION LACK OF PURPOSE FEAR OF SPEAKING & COMPANY	ANGER RAGE SHYNESS LOW CONFIDENCE HIGHLY STRUNG BI-POLAR SLEEP DISORDERS LACK OF INTUITION HALLUCINATIONS [PSYCHIC ABILITIES]	PHOBIAS MELANCHOLIA HIGHLY STRUNG NERVOUS FIDGETY HEAD IN THE 'CLOUDS' [PSYCHIC ABILITIES]
PHYSICAL SYMPTOMS	OSTEO-ARTHRITIS NEPHRITIS CYSTITIS PROSTATITIS LOW BACK PAIN ANKY. SPOND. CHRONIC TIREDNESS	OEDEMA IMPOTENCE LOW LIBIDO MENSTRUAL IMBALANCE CHILLBLAINS LEG ULCERS LETHARGY	ACNE ECZEMA STOMACH ULCER DYSPEPSIA GLANDULAR FEVER CFS CANCER DIABETES HEPATITIS	HEART CONDITIONS POOR CIRCULATION BENIGN TMOURS SCOLIOSIS	SORE THROATS TONSILITIS ASTHMA URTI BRONCHITIS FROZEN SHOULDER COLITIS CONSTIPATION FIBROSITIS	HEADACHES MIGRAINE SINUSITIS CATARRH VERTIGO TINNITUS NEUROLOGICAL EAR CONDITIONS	HEADACHE VERTIGO TINNITUS HYPERTENSION S.A.D. NEUROLOGICAL
MERIDIANS	KIDNEY BLADDER GOVERNING CONCEPTION	SPLEEN PERICARDIUM	STOMACH LIVER	HEART SMALL INTESTINE	LUNG LARGE INTESTINE	GALL BLADDER	TRIPLE ENERGIZER
ENDOCRINE	ADRENALS	OVARIES TESTES	PANCREAS	THYMUS	THYROID PARATHYROID	PITUITARY	PINEAL
SPINAL	COCCYX	L2 - S4	T9 - S1	T4 - T8	C5 - T3	OCC - C4	UPPER CRANIUM
BODY	SPINAL COLUMN KIDNEYS BLADDER BONE	LYMPHATICS REPRODUCTIVE SYSTEM	STOMACH SPLEEN LIVER PANCREAS G.B. SMALL BOWEL	CIRCULATION HEART PNS PERICARDIUM	LUNGS BRONCHUS THROAT LARGE BOWEL	EARS NOSE (L) EYE CNS SNS PNS	CNS (R) EYE
MINOR CHAKRAS	ELBOW KNEE	SPLEEN	SPLEEN	EAR INTERCOSTAL	NAVEL SHOULDER	GROIN CLAVICULAR	HAND FOOT
MAJOR CHAKRA	BASE	SACRAL	SOLAR PLEXUS	HEART	THROAT	BROW	CROWN

Table 1.1 Relationships of the Major Chakras copyright John Cross Publications 2016.

Since completing my acupuncture doctoral thesis in 1987, most of my professional career has been occupied in the clinical practice, teaching and writing about the chakra energy system. The thesis for the British College of Acupuncture dealt with a comparison of traditional Chinese medicine and traditional Ayurvedic and Indian medicine, so the chakras played a big part in it. I wrote about something that no one had done before. I have had the honour of teaching this system to hundreds of practitioners in many parts of the world and in many cases completely changing the pathways in their medical careers. The chakra energy system is vast and composite, and can be used in the treatment of musculo-skeletal, internal organic and emotional/mental conditions. I often compare it, as in the above table, to the Periodic Table of Elements in that there is order and symmetry to it – there is no guess work, 'maybe's' and 'what if's'. What I have attempted to do over the last 30 years is to take the mystique out of a system of healing that was once only linked with yoga, meditation and Hinduism. It goes without saying that my work has been a two edged sword in that it has been met with praise by practitioners and patients alike but also castigated by 'colleagues' who demand that all medicine should be evidence based. I have had to tread a very fine line and at times it has been a struggle. The truth, however, will always out, and to me, the proof of the pudding is in the eating. I care not one fig that this and many other forms of subtle energy medicine isn't accepted by mainstream medicine – it is their loss. I have only ever been interested in the successful treatment of my patients by non-invasive and non-symptomatic means.

Those of you who are well versed in chakra energy will appreciate that the energy 'vibration' differs with each one. The Base chakra, because it is our link with the earth has a very slow vibration, the Sacral chakra is a little higher and the Solar Plexus chakra higher still. The vibrational rate increase exponentially when we reach the Brow and the Crown chakras. When we perform either contact or non-contact healing on the client, we can, with practice, feel the different vibrations. In treatment of chronic energy imbalance for example it is essential that the Base chakra's sluggish energy is stimulated. Likewise, in certain emotional/mental imbalance it may benefit the client if the vibration is lowered. The reason I am emphasising this is that in distant healing the equation of different vibrations in each chakra doesn't enter the equation. This is just one of many advantages of working at a distance. There is, though, quite a difference in the vibrational rate, hence the 'feel' of the four auric bodies that will be described later.

It is possible to analyse and to treat at a distance by using other energy modalities such as the meridian system or to send 'healing' to specific internal organs, acupoints, endocrine glands or even reflexes (reflected points or areas). However, I firmly believe that as the chakra energy system incorporates every physical, emotional and mental attribute in the body, by *only* using this system, you save time and yield better results than with specific targeted healing.

CHAPTER TWO

Dowsing. *Yes/No*. Dowsing from a list. Making an Analysis Chart

Dowsing

Before we look into how to analyse energy imbalance in the major chakras, it is important to mention the topic of dowsing. This book will probably be read by those of you who are already versed in the subject, but there may be several of you who wouldn't have a clue about it. I'll go through the salient points. Firstly, a definition: -

The Dowsing Faculty – is the ability to use the natural sensitivity, which we all possess, that enables us to know things, to seek for and to locate things which we cannot know or do by using cognition, or by learning, or by experience, or by using the five physical senses.

Dowsing has been used for over 6000 years and there are cave paintings at Tassili in the Sahara to substantiate this. One may dowse for minerals, underground water and oil, radiation and Ley lines by using a pendulum, diving rods, hazel twig or even just the fingers. Some folk are so gifted in dowsing that they don't require the tool of a pendulum – they just sense the different vibrations that emanate from the oil or water that they are trying to find. Professional dowsers are employed by oil companies and expert dowsers can find the correct viscosity, the depth, the layers of rock to mine through etc. They save the oil companies a small fortune in cutting out the guess work. It is, though, medical dowsing or radiesthesia that we are interested in. The pendulum is the usual tool of choice and Figure 2.1 shows a selection of some that I have at home. Pendulums may be made from plastic, wood or different types of mineral. The string may be of cotton, string or a metal chain. There is no inherent magic in a pendulum – it is merely an inert tool

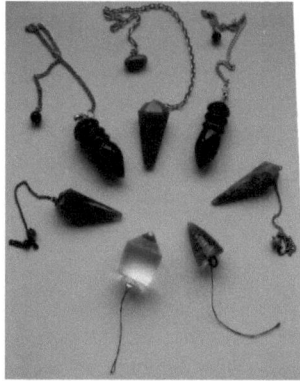

Figure 2.1 Selection of pendulums

My favourite is the chunky clear plastic one at the bottom of the photograph whereas my wife's favourite is the one next to it on the right. There is nothing magical about dowsing and anyone, with training, can do it. It is not spiritual or 'fruitcakey' but a natural phenomenon. We just don't know how it works – but that goes for many things! The pendulum (something allowed to swing) is merely an extension of the arm that in turn is an extension of the brain via the central nervous system. **Dowsing works through thought.** It is extremely important that this phrase is understood. It is your own thoughts that guides the movement of the pendulum. Thought originates in the Mental Body of the aura, more often called 'Thought Forms'. When we think there has to be a reaction as it is a form of energy. Two truisms are 'Thought is Energy' and 'Movement follows Thought'. When we think something, there has to be a reaction – I guess a little bit like Newton's first Law of Motion. Dowsing through thought is the response to constructive questions that you ask of the client (or the representative of the client in the Witness).

Yes/No

It is essential that all questions asked of the Witness *must* have a *yes/no* response. You cannot ask any question that does not comply with this. It is therefore not possible – or ethical- to ask what numbers are going to win the lottery or which horse will win the 3.30 race - you will just be given a 'gobbledegook' reply. We each have our own *Yes* and *No* response and it is important that this is known before you do anything. To ascertain your response, sit comfortably in a chair with your shoulders relaxed and your pendulum in your prime hand with the string/cotton between your thumb and forefinger. Start the pendulum swinging in a front and back movement i.e. between 6 and 12 o'clock. Keep this swing direction going for a few seconds without any extraneous thoughts in your head. Then ask silently 'What is my *Yes*'? The pendulum will start to move in the direction that is positive for you. Then wilfully swing the pendulum in a front/back movement again and then ask silently 'What is my *No*?' The pendulum will then move in the direction that indicates your negative response. It is a good discipline to ask each and every time before you work. The answer should always be the same though. My *Yes* is a clockwise direction circle and my *No* is a 45-degree straight line swing to the left. My wife's are completely different. I am not of the school of thought that dowsing should commence with a still and non-swinging pendulum, as in attempting to dowse the gender of an unborn child. Pendulums are meant to swing!

Dowsing from a list

So as to test out the *yes/no* phenomenon with your pendulum, you can make various lists. When I teach this topic to delegates who have no experience in dowsing I always start with teaching how to dowse from a list first before we explain about making a dowsing chart, as it is a good discipline. You may write down a list of foods, non-foods etc. that you think there may be a sensitive or an allergic reaction, or write down a list of vertebral levels, internal organs, joints etc. where you feel there may be problems. You may do this with some of your hair or that of a family member (with their permission). It isn't the most straightforward of disciplines to ask questions about oneself as you are too close so it's best to start with someone else. The technique of doing this will be discussed later in the chapter.

Before you start dowsing

It is extremely important that you dowse whilst you are relaxed and well – never dowse when you are feeling unwell or feel that you cannot concentrate. It is also important that you are meant to do what you are doing – be it analysis or healing. Therefore, ask a silent question before you start 'is it OK to analyse/send healing to so and so'. This is mandatory and should never be skipped. The other important thing to do is to ground yourself. This is just being comfortable by placing your feet firmly on the floor – not with legs crossed or feet off the ground. Some dowsers (me included) will also 'protect' themselves from any extraneous energies that may well be around. I am not talking about demons, goblins and angels here, but protecting yourself from any perverse energy manifestations in the room, such as electro-magnetic forces from an electric clock, computer etc. We shall mention further aspects of grounding yourself in the next chapter.

General to Specific questioning

If you have ever used Teletext or the red button (in the UK), through your television, you will know that you commence with the various genres of News, Sport, Weather, Finance etc. Once you are into, say, Sport you find another list that includes all the individual sports such as football, cricket, F1, rugby etc. Then you open the page that you want and are confronted with another set of headings. Finally, you will reach the specific page that gives you the information you want. So it is with dowsing – you start with the general and work down to the specific. This is fundamentally important. Say, for instance, you want to ascertain why your client is having pain in the spine. You firstly ask if the pain is in the spine as a whole – *Yes*. Then you ask if it is the thoracic spine – *Yes*. Then you go down a list (or just ask) which of the thoracic vertebral levels are affected. Now you know which one is the culprit, you ask many other questions (all of which have to have a *yes/no* answer) of the individual vertebra dependent upon your anatomical knowledge.

I.F.

Students of mine will know what the letters 'I' and 'F' stand for. In actual practice the 'F' comes before the 'I', but it's easier to remember IF than FI. They stand for *Focus* and *Intention*. Focus means that you concentrate ONLY on the task in hand without letting your mind wander to other things – you think only of the client and the Witness in front of you. When the client is in the room, you concentrate one hundred percent on them, so why not with distance healing? Intention merely means that you think about the action you are taking. In the situation of treating the client on couch if, say, you are attempting to energy balance between two acupoints using conductive acupressure, at the same time that you have your fingers on the points you *think* about energy movement. Your thought forms are hugely important. So it is with distance analysis and healing – you think about every single action that you do at the same time that they are being performed.

Energy Follows Thought

You now know the importance and power of your thought forms – what you think is crucial in all forms of healing, but especially in distance analysis and healing. You will have noticed the last two words in the title of this book – My Way! This means exactly what it says on the tin. This book is about what I do, and have done for many years, and not based on anyone else's ideas. There are many aspects to dowsing and several different interpretations of how to perform it practically. So below is the nuts and bolts of my style of dowsing – firstly from a list and secondly from a chart.

Yes/No from a list

Test your *yes/no*. I know that it will usually never change but it gets you in the groove for the dowsing session. Make sure that you are in a fit state to dowse, also that you are meant to be dowsing over the particular Witness – test by asking *yes/no*. Do this each and every time. Occasionally I have been given the 'no' in each category – for whatever reason.

Start the pendulum swinging up and down (6 o'clock and 12 o 'clock) – this is usually a neutral swing. With a list of, say, the seven major chakras in front of you make sure that you have silently asked the question e.g. "is there an imbalance in the Base chakra" just before you focus your eyes on the words 'Base chakra' on your list. The pendulum should immediately give you either a *yes* or *no* response. You may augment this with pointing at the words with your non pendulum holding hand. So with words, thought and gesture you are focussing on the subject.

Once you have the answer, either remember it, put your pendulum down and write the answer with a pencil, or speak into a Dictaphone (my choice). Then start the up and down swing and focus on the next question associated with the next word on the list.

You may also ask *yes/no* questions using a chart by focussing the gaze and pointing to a word in the chart. However, usually dowsing from a chart is different to the *yes/no* with a list.

Drawing a chart

Charts are usually drawn on A4 paper. You may purchase a readymade one or make your own. The following is how to make your own from scratch. Below is a typical skeleton framework with which you can complete – Figure 2.2 refers. As you can see, all you need is an A4 piece of paper, a compass and ruler. There are seven sections on my chart to represent various aspects of the seven major chakras. The Witness (hair sample) is placed at the lower concave area. Numbers 1-10 are placed around this as this is a good way of ascertaining the energy levels/prognosis when asked - Figure 2.3 refers. The skeleton chart here shows just six segments where you write in various associations of the major chakras, although you may have as many as you like – the size of the paper you use is the determining factor. Please note that these three are not in scale with each other. It is important that each section is roughly the same size as its neighbour and that there is enough room in each box to place salient words corresponding to the chakra and system. The systems may be written under the left hand side of the chart, but this is not essential. It will be fun to create your own unique chart. Many of my students have done just that, and I have been amazed with their ingenious efforts.

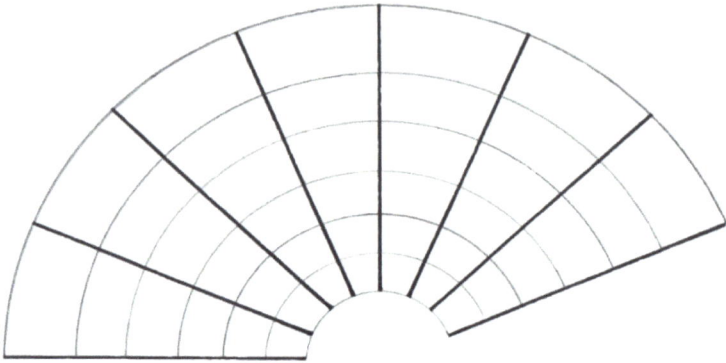

Figure 2.2 Skeleton Chart

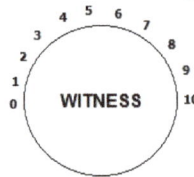

Figure 2.3 Witness area with 1-10 numbers surrounding

Figure 2.4 shows the first segment with the names of the major chakras in order. I usually find that colour coordinating them with the standard chakra colours of red, orange, yellow, green, blue, indigo and violet helps with the focus and intention.

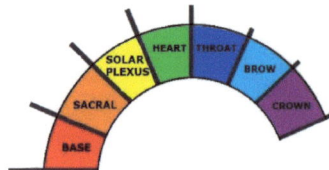

Figure 2.4 First segment of chart showing major chakras

The remainder of the segments may comprise of the associated minor chakras, internal organs, endocrine glands, spinal levels, meridians and emotions. Of course you may also use this template as a complete dowsing tool that could include such titles as prognosis, aetiology, peripheral joints, homoeopathic/herbal, and general treatment protocols. Figure 2.5 shows the above skeleton chart completed to just six relationships of the major chakras. It is a help or guide for you – what you *should* do is to make your own. This is not because I don't want to spoon feed you – I've spent the last 4 decades doing just that with seminar delegates! It is because if you create your own chart it will be YOURS and your conscious and, what is more important, your sub conscious brain will know and comprehend it.

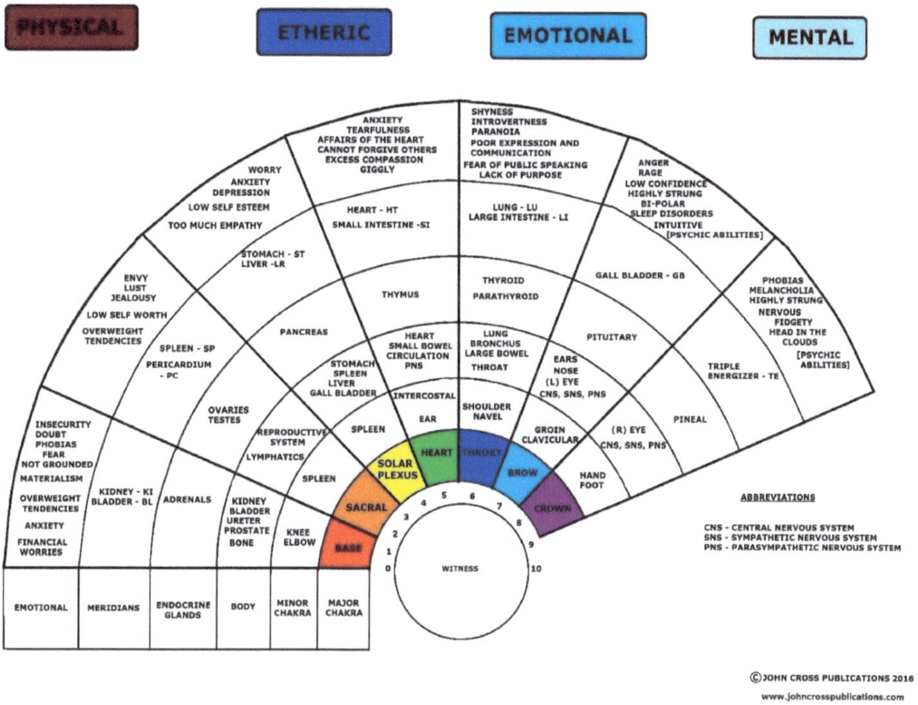

PHYSICAL   ETHERIC   EMOTIONAL   MENTAL

Figure 2.5 Chakra chart for analysis

Dowsing from your chart

The Witness is placed upon the circle. Dowsing from a chart is quite different to dowsing from a list using the *yes/no* response. This is because you don't necessarily ask questions that have a *yes/no* reply. Questions are asked that will make the pendulum swing in the direction of the reply. For instance – you may ask which major chakra is in need of healing – the pendulum then swings in the direction of the chakra on the chart. You may then ask what the general energy quality of the chakra in need of healing is. The pendulum will then swing to one of the numbers on the witness circle. This will give you a base reading

11

that will be checked after you have sent some healing. This is something that needs to be practised over and over again until you feel that you have mastered it. This will only occur if you follow the guidance given earlier in this chapter of giving focus and intention to the task in hand. Always remember that someone has entrusted you to help them and it is a great privilege so to do. Being sloppy will not produce the desired effects and you owe it to your client and yourself to give one hundred percent.

How does dowsing from a chart work?

A simple answer would be 'I don't know', and it would be truthful. I guess that no one can proffer a rationale behind this phenomenon. We have to give all the credit to our amazing central nervous system and in particular the sub conscious brain. I have carried out my own style of research over the last few years in that I changed the style and type of analytical chart I used. Once each one had been drawn and studied with my conscious brain, it seems that the unconscious brain accepted the information immediately and responded to give the same correct answers each time. So it doesn't matter which 'directional' question you ask, the pendulum will swing in the correct direction regardless of where in each chart the answer resides.

The next chapter will deal with analytical dowsing in detail.

CHAPTER THREE
Analysis of the Major Chakras at the Physical, Etheric, Emotional and Mental levels.

You now have the basic knowledge to be able to do a full analytical assessment of your client's chakra energy system. You will require total concentration, focus and intention in order to be the expert that you want to be. The chart uses a combination of the *yes/no* answer, where you know what your *yes* and *no* swings are, and where you ask a non *yes/no* reply and the pendulum swings towards the correct answer. You have to keep switching from one mode to the other in order to do it well.

The Witness

It has already been stated that the Witness represents the client in that the vibrational rate that it holds is exactly the same as the whole person. I personally like to use a lock of hair, but a recent photograph will do. Rarely do we get involved in blood spots these days. It must be placed in a small plastic bag by the client with no outside contamination. The plastic container should fit within the circle so that it's possible to read the numbers encircling it.

Preparation

You should be comfortably seated with the chart/Witness in front of you. You may either write your answers down or use a Dictaphone with your non dowsing hand. The problem with writing things down as you go is that the pendulum hand is usually your dominant hand and you have to keep putting the pendulum down to write. Once you are ready to commence make sure that you have no outside interferences and that your mobile phone is switched off. You cannot dowse and listen to your favourite music at the same time!! As stated before you may take a few seconds to 'ground' and protect yourself with your feet on the floor. I usually say a short mantra or imagine my head surrounded by a goldfish bowl so there are no extraneous energies entering my psyche. This is more important in the healing mode than in analysis mode. As you may have noticed I have purposely omitted the 'physical' symptoms on the analysis chart above. This is because these will already be known to you as the client's symptoms. It is up to you to decide the *cause* of the symptoms and which chakra level is in a state of imbalance.

Order of analytical assessment

1. **Ascertain the main energy imbalance and at which level**
   Start the pendulum swinging in a neutral direction. Then ask in turn if the main imbalance lies in the Physical, Etheric, Emotional or Mental Body. You ask 'Is the main imbalance in the Physical Body?' and get a *yes/no* reply for this. Then proceed through the other three. Once you know the main imbalance you may calculate which one has secondary or a lesser imbalance – and so on.

2. **Gauge the energetic value of each chakra.**
   Commence with the Base chakra and proceed in turn to the Crown chakra. You simply ask the question 'what is the general energetic value of the .... chakra?' The pendulum will swing to the direction of the correct number around the witness circle. Anything that reads over 8 is usually very good and no need for intervention. Readings between 5 and 7 are borderline of requiring treatment or healing later on. Anything under 5 indicates that the chakra is in a poor state of balance (congested) and will require treatment or healing. There may be anything up to 3 chakras with a rating of under 5 and they will all need looking at. Each of the chakras that showed up to be congested need to be analysed specifically in order that treatment and healing may be specifically tuned. I shall cover all four scenarios below but in practice you will only need to analyse the main and secondary ones.

3. **Physical Body Energy Analysis**.
   The first stage is to analyse the PHYSICAL body. This is the body that we see and the one that houses the symptoms. Although you are interested in the client's symptoms, in practical terms you are more interested in the energetic state of the subtler bodies, as it is those that gave the symptoms within the physical body in the first place, unless they were caused by accident or injury. Always start in-depth analysis on the Base chakra – this is because it is *the* one that is always in a state of imbalance in chronic illness. The Base chakra represents the foundation on which the others sit. Comparing it to the basement of a block of flats would be a good analogy. To do this, start the pendulum swinging up and down and firstly ask 'what is the energetic value of the Base chakra' (a confirmation of what you had done earlier). You must switch your thoughts now to PHYSICAL body mode. It will help if you stare at the word on the top left of the page. You must also keep concentrating on the words Base chakra. Now you ask *yes/no* questions on all the aspects about the Base chakra and your pendulum will give you a *yes/no* reply. You may ask if the minor chakras of Knee and Elbow are also energetically low – if the answer is *no*, you proceed to the next stage, if the answer is *yes* you then ask the energy quality of each in turn. This is where you must be ready in an instance to switch the pendulum mode between *yes/no* and allowing the pendulum to give you an answer. You then ask if the associated body areas are energetically low – take the bladder, kidney, ureter, prostate and bone individually. The word 'bone' here relates to anything related to bony inflammation, such as arthritis. You may also ask about the spinal levels – although the spine isn't represented in this particular analysis chart. Proceed to ask about the associated endocrine gland (adrenals) and meridians. All the replies have to be logged. You then come to the 'emotional' box. This may sound a bit crazy in that you asking about the physical aspect of the Base chakra – but remember you are looking for the aetiology (cause) of the imbalance. This box is probably the most important and must be done very carefully. It goes without saying that the words in each box are mine – there are very many alternative aspects – it is only the size of the box that is the limiting factor as to how many emotional aspects of each chakra you write down. You don't necessarily give each of the emotional aspects a 1-10 score, it is sufficient just to ask a *yes/no* question for each.

4. **Etheric Body Energy Analysis.**
   The next stage is to assess the ETHERIC aspect of the Base chakra. The word is derived from 'ether' meaning the state between matter and energy. It consists of a network of fine tubular threadlike channels commonly known as *nadis*, and these in turn are related to the cerebrospinal fluid, endocrine glands and the autonomic nervous system. The etheric body is a field of energy that underlies every cell and atom of the physical body by permeating every part of it. Readings at the etheric level tend to be similar to the physical body. When there is a large discrepancy it usually means that the imbalance has originated within the physical body and not the usual way round of energy imbalance originating at the mental level. This could be eating too much fat, sugar or other similar foods that clog the system. Similarly, smoking will affect the etheric Throat chakra. Proceed in the exact same fashion as per the Physical body. Don't forget to repeatedly stare at the word ETHERIC at the top of the page.

5. **Emotional Body Energy Analysis.**
   The next stage is the assessment of the EMOTIONAL body of the Base chakra. The Emotional (or Astral) aura deals with our feelings. We are bombarded on a daily basis by stimuli of one sort or another from internal and external sources. The vast majority of physical body imbalances (symptoms) are derived from an aggravation to the emotional body caused by constant negative emotions such as anger or fear from within or by the filtering of 'thought forms' from the Mental body. This auric field is probably the most important, active, and yet the most complicated, in the subtle body. Proceed as before only staring at the word EMOTIONAL at the top of the page.

6. **Mental Body Energy Analysis.**
   The final stage is the assessment of the MENTAL body of the Base chakra. This extremely fine and subtle body deals with thoughts and mental processes, sometimes called 'thought forms'. In simple language, when we think, this is the region where our thoughts are originated. What we think affects us and those with whom we come into contact. If our natures are engendering, positive and helpful and we direct lots of lovely thoughts to other living creatures, we feel well within. In contrast, if we show negativity, hatred, pessimism, grief, sorrow or depressive tendencies, these are eventually reflected in our physical body make up. Please remember the adage 'we become what we think'. It is said that we are totally responsible for our own health, or as much of it as we have been granted at conception and birth. Proceed as before and this time keep staring at the word MENTAL at the top right of the page.

When you have completed the Base chakra analysis proceed to the next chakra that initially gave you the lowest reading. For example - if a person has a history of chest problems possibly coupled with bowel symptoms – the Throat chakra would certainly be in a state of energy imbalance and would be the main one to analyse after the Base. You may need to analyse all seven but this is rare – usually four would be the maximum. The above looks a little daunting at first but practice makes perfect, as long as you keep obeying the basic rules of focus and intention you cannot go wrong. The main trap when you start analytical dowsing is to assume the answer – especially if you know the client well. Never pre judge anything and try to stay aloof – never let your own feelings enter the fray. This is particularly important when you are analysing members of your own family – even the family pet. It is, though, sometimes impossible to stay aloof as, try as you may, your own feelings come to the fore.

CHAPTER FOUR

Distance Healing at the Etheric, Emotional and Mental levels

If you have carried out your analysis correctly and have tabulated your findings, you are now in a position to carry out distance healing. Healing always was and always will be an emotive subject. The word simply means 'to make whole', but as we all know- it is much more than that. It does not mean 'cure' and none of us is in a position to state that curing takes place. There are many theories as to how distance healing works but the bottom line is that we just don't know for certain. The only thing I can state for certain is that it seems to work. A few of the ideas that surround it are: -

- **Prayer.** Prayer for the sick either from an individual or a group has been practised in most religions for thousands of years. In Christianity it remains one of the 'gifts of the Spirit' and it is thought that healing occurs through the power of the Holy Spirit. Other religions such as Islam, Judaism, Hinduism, Buddhism and Shamanism each have their own interpretations. Prayer can be very powerful and represents a huge source of comfort for the recipient.
- **Reiki.** Traditional reiki teaches distant healing as well as contact healing. This is performed by the interpretation of symbols that allows 'reiki energy' to be sent over the ether to the client.
- **Thought.** Some people do not require the ritual discipline of a religious faith or reiki in order to send healing. It is performed purely through the power of thought. The maxim 'energy follows thought' is very important. It must, however, be performed in a structured way in order that the recipient gains some benefit.
- **Scientific interpretation.** Recent discoveries in quantum physics has shown that time is not fixed either in direction or viscosity. It shows that everything is happening at once, there is no past and no future, only the present. Because of this there is no such thing as linear distance and that everything is linked. It does seem amazing to me that what the Shamans and other traditional healers have instinctively known for centuries is now being 'proved' by science. On a personal note, though, I take some of the quantum physics rationale with a huge pinch of salt. When a so called science tells us that there is no such thing as reality – and it is accepted because the boffins have decreed it so – I despair (or is it me?) We shall see what further revelations bring us.
- **Radionics.** Another type of distance healing is to use a radionics 'black box'. This works by the radionics practitioner placing the witness on a metal plate on a black box containing several dials. He/she then turns each of the dials to the number representing the vibrational 'rate' that is to be 'beamed' to the client, either for the whole energy system (called the personal general rate (PGR)) or to individual organs and system that each have a specific vibrational rate. The theory is one of energy patterns and identifying the electrodynamic patterns emitted by matter of all kinds. I used radionics in my dim and distant past but found it was too 'mechanical'. I found out that I could use my own style of radionics by merely using a chart and my own thoughts and discounting the box. As an aside here, I was in attendance at the Radionics Association conference in Poole in the early 1980's when David Tansley (the author of many excellent books) announced that he too had discounted the magic box and that all you needed was 'thought'. It made a few of the radionics doyens cough, splutter and faint in the aisles, but vindicated my work entirely.
- **My own theory.** You may probably have heard of Schumann's Resonance. In 1952 the German Scientist Professor W.O. Schumann of Munich University discovered that there are electromagnetic standing waves in the atmosphere within the cavity formed by the earth's surface and the ionosphere. He found a mean reading of 7.83 cycles per second (cps) or hertz. Subsequently the research made by Dr. Herbert Konig (Schumann's successor at Munich) found that the mean vibrational rate of the earth (7.83 cps) was equivalent to the brain wave frequency at the level between the alpha and theta waves – called the alpha-theta frequency. To put this in perspective, the brain wave frequency of the awake and alert person (beta) is 13 cps upwards. The more relaxed

state of alpha is between 8 and 13 cps. Theta state of drowsiness is 4-8 cps and the sleep state of delta waves is below 4 cps. I have found over the past 35 years that a 'oneness' between the practitioner and patient (or healer and client) occurs at the Schumann's resonance of 7.83 cps. I have stated on numerous occasions that healing cannot occur until both healer and client has reached this vibrational state. Dr. Cyril Smith, now retired and late of Salford University U.K. and author of scores of books and hundreds of articles on vibrational frequency, postulated the frequencies of many acupuncture points, including the ones that are the physical placements of the major chakras. He found that the frequency of Heart chakra at both Con 17 (front) and at Gov 10 (between T6-7) in the centre of the spine had a frequency range between 7.68 and 7.92 cps. It doesn't take a genius to realise that the frequency of the very centre of our being is the same as the natural vibrational frequency of our planet. Therefore, if we send healing with unconditional love, originating from our Heart chakra, we realign the client's energy disharmony into one of harmony with their surroundings and environment and thus allow their body to commence self-healing.

NEGATIVE QUALITIES	INSECURITY DOUBT PHOBIAS FEAR NOT GROUNDED ANXIETY FINANCE WORRIES DWELLS ON MATERIALISM OVERWEIGHT TENDENCIES	JEALOUSY ENVY LUST LOW SELF WORTH NYMPHOMANIA OVERWEIGHT TENDENCIES TATS	DEPRESSION WORRY ANXIETY LOW SELF ESTEEM TOO MUCH EMPATHY	TEARFULNESS ANXIETY AFFAIRS OF THE HEART CANNOT FORGIVE OTHERS EXCESS EMPATHY & COMPASSION GIGGLY	SHYNESS INTROVERTNESS PARANOIA POOR EXPRESSION & COMMUNICATION LACK OF PURPOSE FEAR OF SPEAKING & COMPANY	ANGER RAGE SHYNESS LOW CONFIDENCE HIGHLY STRUNG BI-POLAR LACK OF INTUITION HALLUCINATIONS [PSYCHIC ABILITIES]	PHOBIAS MELANCHOLIA HIGHLY STRUNG NERVOUS FIDGETY HEAD IN THE 'CLOUDS' [PSYCHIC ABILITIES]
PHYSICAL SYMPTOMS	OSTEO-ARTHRITIS NEPHRITIS CYSTITIS PROSTATITIS LOW BACK PAIN ANKY. SPOND. CHRONIC TIREDNESS	OEDEMA IMPOTENCE LOW LIBIDO MENSTRUAL IMBALANCE CHILLBLAINS LEG ULCERS LETHARGY	ACNE ECZEMA STOMACH ULCER DYSPEPSIA GLANDULAR FEVER CFS CANCER DIABETES HEPATITIS	HEART CONDITIONS POOR CIRCULATION BENIGN TMOURS SCOLIOSIS	SORE THROATS TONSILITIS ASTHMA URTI BRONCHITIS FROZEN SHOULDER COLITIS CONSTIPATION FIBROSITIS	HEADACHES MIGRAINE SINUSITIS CATARRH VERTIGO TINNITUS NEUROLOGICAL EAR CONDITIONS	HEADACHE VERTIGO TINNITUS HYPERTENSION S.A.D. NEUROLOGICAL
MERIDIANS	KIDNEY BLADDER GOVERNING CONCEPTION	SPLEEN PERICARDIUM	STOMACH LIVER	HEART SMALL INTESTINE	LUNG LARGE INTESTINE	GALL BLADDER	TRIPLE ENERGIZER
ENDOCRINE	ADRENALS	OVARIES TESTES	PANCREAS	THYMUS	THYROID PARATHYROID	PITUITARY	PINEAL
SPINAL	COCCYX	L2 - S4	T9 - S1	T4 - T8	C5 - T3	OCC - C4	UPPER CRANIUM
BODY	SPINAL COLUMN KIDNEYS BLADDER BONE	LYMPHATICS REPRODUCTIVE SYSTEM	STOMACH SPLEEN LIVER PANCREAS G.B. SMALL BOWEL	CIRCULATION HEART PNS PERICARDIUM	LUNGS BRONCHUS THROAT LARGE BOWEL	EARS NOSE (L) EYE CNS SNS PNS	CNS (R) EYE
MINOR CHAKRAS	ELBOW KNEE	SPLEEN	SPLEEN	EAR INTERCOSTAL	NAVEL SHOULDER	GROIN CLAVICULAR	HAND FOOT
MAJOR CHAKRA	BASE	SACRAL	SOLAR PLEXUS	HEART	THROAT	BROW	CROWN

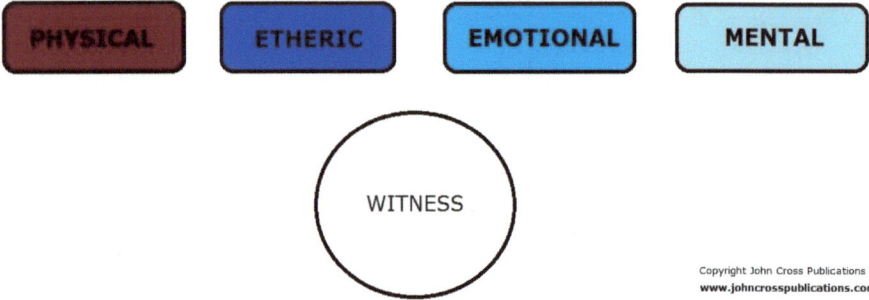

PHYSICAL   ETHERIC   EMOTIONAL   MENTAL

WITNESS

Figure 4.1 Distance Healing Chart using the Major Chakras

Preparation for distance healing

Some of this has already been stated but it does no harm to reaffirm because it is all important. Try not to cut corners or walk before you can run – you will not get the desired results. Below is a nominal list to which you should adhere.

- Gain permission from the recipient. Never send healing to anyone without their explicit permission. In the case of babies, minors or animals, seek the permission of the parent, guardian or owner. Don't take it for granted that because you have been requested to do an analysis that you also have permission to send healing.
- Never send healing if you are unwell – by that I mean that if you feel too tired or that you cannot concentrate for more than a few minutes.
- Make it part of your weekly routine. I usually have set days and times where I carry out my distance healing and I only vary from that in an emergency. You need to have some 'me time' and not become a slave of your work – stress will ensue if you do!
- I do not think it is important that the recipient or client knows the exact time that healing is to take place. I am not one of those who thinks the client should be lying down relaxed at a specific time. It is a fact that some clients know instinctively when healing is occurring but generally they do not. This type of healing is not instantaneous 'zap' healing. It makes changes to their aura in a very subtle way, eventually creating changes within their physical bodies.
- Before you start the distance healing session, make sure that you are cocooned in your room with no outside noise or interference (switch off the mobile phone) and make sure that you will not be disturbed.
- Grounding yourself is important in that as we are dealing with very subtle energies we should ground ourselves through the Base chakra to the earth. One of my favourite sayings is that 'you can have your head in the clouds so long as you have your feet on the ground'. I place my feet on the floor and imagine myself rooted to the earth. I also imagine a goldfish bowl around my head so I remain protected at all times. You may also say a silent mantra or prayer and some practitioners think that this helps.

The Distance Healing Chart

Figure 4.1 shows the distance healing chart I use. Please study it in detail. Although it is the one I use, as I stated when describing the distance analysis chart, it is vital that you make up your own – to your own requirements. The Witness is placed in the Witness circle – please note that as we are not analysing it is not necessary to have numbers around the circle. Above that are the auric bodies to enable you to focus. Above the individual colour coded chakras are their many associations – these are written down to serve as an aide de memoir. Please note that you no longer require your pendulum. Pendulums are necessary in analysis but *not* in the healing mode.

My Technique

- You already have the results of the analysis and the healing is directed to those areas that require it. You may, for example, have found an energy imbalance in the Etheric aspect of the Base chakra, the Emotional aspect of the Throat chakra and the Mental aspect of the Solar Plexus chakra and it is those that you address in order of severity. Having said that, the Base chakra will always take precedence. Place the Witness on the circle and follow the preparation as above.
- **Initial Moves.** With complete focus make circular movements with one or both hands above the Witness about 2.5 cms (1") for about one minute or so. This is so as to make contact (or rather non-

17

contact) with the Witness and to 'build up' the energy matrix around the Witness. As you circle the hands (mainly with the finger ends) you will notice a sensation of warmth that slowly increases in intensity. As the warmth increases and you feel that you have made 'contact', that is the time to start the specific healing. This initial move is very important. It is much like non-contact conductive healing that is carried out around an area of chronicity (yin) directly on your patient. If, for example, you are giving non-contact healing to an arthritic hip you would build up the energy around the hip by performing circular (clockwise or anti-clockwise, it doesn't matter) movements about an inch away from the physical body. You notice that a degree of warmth appears under your fingers and the patient will inform you that they feel heat and a relaxation of the tissues (that will eventually lead to pain relief). So it is no different to perform this on a Witness. It helps in the focus if you silently say that you are building up the energy.

THE PHYSICAL BODY

Overview

The Physical Body is the one that we as therapists see, touch, pummel, stroke, heat up or stick needles into. Looking at the person from a purely esoteric viewpoint, the Physical or Dense Body has very little significance. The most important aspect of the Physical Body is that it gives us the signs and symptoms of energy imbalance. Symptoms are golden pearls of information that are used by the practitioner in considering the cause of dis-ease. Some readers may be surprised that healing can be sent directly to the Physical Body when, as we know, healing is transmitted directly to the subtler bodies in order to help the symptoms that are merely housed within the physical body. I was taught just that, but after experimenting for a couple of years, I found that I had beneficial results when directing healing directly at the physical body. Remember that the physical is also made up of energy (as is everything) – it is just that it appears to resonate at a lower and more sluggish level than the subtle bodies.

Healing

To send healing to the Physical Body the hands are kept perfectly still at about the same distance away from the Witness as the initial moves – approximately 2.5 cms (1 inch). Touching the Witness does not enhance this healing mode so stay about 2.5 cms away. With your fingers in situ take your gaze towards the **PHYSICAL** body box and think 'PHYSICAL BODY' as you do it. You then direct your gaze and focus to the chakra and the part of the body that you wish to send healing. If, for example, you wish to send healing towards the gall bladder organ, you stare at **PHYSICAL** for a few seconds, then the **SOLAR PLEXUS** chakra (colour coded yellow) and take the eyes up to the gall bladder in the 'Body' list. It always helps to actually say (aloud or silently) what you are attempting with your thoughts – energy follows thought! With your focus totally on the physical body and the body area concerned, now say any statement with which you are comfortable in order to facilitate the healing process. It could be 'I am sending healing to the ......' or 'Allow healing to take place on ......' or 'the ...... is being made whole' or whatever you are comfortable with. You are constantly focussed on the words **PHYSICAL** and **SOLAR PLEXUS** as well as the target area.

Sensations under the fingers

With physical body healing, the sensations you have initially is one of warmth. As the seconds tick by, there will be a kind of buffering or resistance between the fingers and the Witness – this doesn't always happen but mostly does. This sensation lasts for as long as the healing is necessary and is a signal that healing needs to continue. When the healing has achieved its target, the resistance sensation will suddenly disappear and it will feel much lighter, yet still warm, under the fingers. That is the sign that the healing has been achieved. It may be accompanied by you taking a deep breath or sighing – this is an automatic reaction from the autonomic nervous system. As soon as this sensation occurs you may proceed with any other physical body healing.

THE ETHERIC BODY

Overview

The Etheric Body is the first subtle body that many people, not just clairvoyants, can see. It is possible for everyone to detect the etheric body with training. There are actually two aspects of the Etheric Body namely the Physical-Etheric and the Etheric-Emotional. The Physical -Etheric Body consists of a network of fine tubular threadlike channels known as the nadis which in turn is related to the autonomic nervous system, the endocrine system and cerebro-spinal fluid. The outer edge of the Etheric Body is approximately ten centimetres (four inches). The main functions of this body are to act a receiver, assimilator and transmitter of vital force via the chakras. It represents a vast clearing house of energy from inside-out and outside-in. Some of the more esoteric tomes state that the etheric is a direct replica of the physical, containing internal organs etc. Although Etheric Body imbalance can give symptoms to any part of the body, it is the fluid systems that are most associated with it, so we generally think of the blood circulation, lymphatic circulation, central nervous system, autonomic nervous system, endocrine glands (hormones) and cerebro-spinal fluid when directing our healing. I generally treat the circulation of the meridian system through the Emotional Body.

Healing

To send healing to the Etheric Body, following the initial moves of building the energy (as described above), very slowly move the hands, with focus on the finger ends, in a circle no higher than 10 cms (4") above the Witness. This could be in a clockwise or anti-clockwise direction. You will now be in the Etheric body of the Witness, which represents the client as a whole. Take your gaze to the **ETHERIC** box and dwell there for a few moments. Then direct your eyes to the major chakra involved – for instance if you want to send healing to the thyroid gland, this would be the **THROAT** chakra. For the length of the healing (it could last from a few seconds to a couple of minutes) keep your focus on the **ETHERIC** box and the part of the body to which you are directing the healing. Don't forget to say out loud what you are attempting with your hands – very important!

Sensations under the fingers

When sending healing through the Etheric Body, the fingers will appear to be quite warm throughout the duration. Whilst the fingers gently circle up to 10 cms. above the Witness (usually about 7 cms or 3 inches) you may find one or two 'hot spots'. The hot spots may feel extra warm or give a tingling or buzzing sensation. If you find just one of these hot spots. Keep one of your hands perfectly still at this place. If there are two hot spots, direct the fingertips of each hand over each and then keep the fingers very still. The signal that the healing has completed is that the sensation suddenly disappears and fizzles out and you may have the autonomic reaction as described before. You will already have noticed that working in the Etheric Body feels much lighter and subtler than the Physical Body.

THE EMOTIONAL BODY

Overview

The Emotional Body varies from 10cms. (4 inches) to approximately 25 cms (10 inches) away from the physical body. It is, without a doubt, the most important and most used when it comes to healing, either directly on the client or at a distance. In the Emotional or Astral Body, multitudes of changes are constantly taking place, even if one is not aware of this fact. We are literally bombarded by stimuli of one sort or another from external and internal sources. The main function of this body is to act as a filter, similar to the etheric body, of stimuli coming toward the physical body from the mental body and those stimuli created within the physical body. The changes in our emotions can ultimately lead to alteration and symptoms within the physical body. It is now perceived that the vast majority of physical symptoms occur due to aggravation within the Emotional Body. This aggravation (for want of a better word) is caused by negative emotions such as anger or fear within the Emotional Body or the filtering of 'thought forms' from within the Mental Body. When a person exhibits negative emotional feelings, even for a short while, the destructive potential created within the Emotional Body eventually affects that area of the physical body to which it is associated. A simple example from hundreds of scenarios would be someone who has shyness and the inability to express their feelings easily would give rise to symptoms in the neck, shoulders and large bowel as the Throat chakra would be affected.

Healing

Following the initial building up of the energy field around the Witness as previously described, take the hands no higher than 25 cms or 10 inches (with a mean distance of approximately 6 inches) away from the Witness and, with total concentration, commence a gentle sweep with one or both hands in a circle about the size of a side plate (approximately 9 inches diameter) with the Witness in the centre of the circle. You may take the hands clockwise or anti-clockwise – it doesn't matter. I always commence at the top of the circle and proceed in a clockwise direction all the way around and back to the top. Once at the top I then gently feel around the centre of the circle. If you can equate this circle as being a large clock – you would commence the sweep at 12 o'clock and take the hand around the clock visiting 3 o'clock, 6 o'clock and 9 o'clock before returning to 12 o'clock. The clock correlation is very important as you will know exactly where in the clock different sensations are picked up with the fingers. The sensations vary enormously form person to person. The area that requires your attention may show itself by a 'fizzing', 'buzzing' or even 'water trickling' sensation. It is very important that you remember where in the clock this sensation is felt. Let us imagine that your previous analysis has given you an Emotional Body imbalance within the Sacral chakra. So in the healing mode your emphasis will be on the **EMOTIONAL** box and the **SACRAL** Chakra (colour coded orange). Now let us assume that you found an altered sensation at, say, 3 o'clock. In the Emotional Body, any imbalance found has to be energy balanced with the associated major chakra – in this case it is the Throat chakra. The way I do this is to keep either one or both hands over the 3 o'clock area and keep transferring my eyes between the **SACRAL** Chakra and the **THROAT** Chakra boxes, whilst at the same time saying out loud or silently 'I am balancing energy between the Throat chakra and Sacral chakra' OR 'I am supporting the Sacral chakra with its partner' OR 'make these two areas as one'. The idea is to imagine that the two areas are blending together into one harmonious entity. When this has occurred (see below) you can now say 'I am sending healing to the Sacral chakra' or such like as you did for the Etheric Body.

Sensations under the fingers

This body is even more subtle than the Etheric, so the sensations you feel are different. They will feel light and airy and not so heated as the previous two. As stated before, you may feel all manner of different sensations. The most common is a slight electric shock tingle. This sensation will change once the healing has been positively completed to one of warmth and the tingling will go. It is always a good thing to scan again once you feel you have achieved the healing as a second site may have been masked. Proceed as before.

Below, as a reminder are the coupled major chakras

Coupled Major Chakras

Base chakra is coupled with both the **Crown** and **Brow** chakras

Sacral chakra is coupled with the **Throat** chakra

Solar Plexus chakra is coupled with the **Heart** chakra

Interpretation of Energy Imbalance of the Chakras at the Etheric/Emotional level

As stated before, the auric chakra is in the shape of an ice cream cone. Looking down on the auric chakra, clairvoyants have described concentric circles within each that differ in number depending on the chakra. For example, the Base chakra has four whilst the Brow chakra has ninety-six. This are not so important in distance healing. The very important part though is that the chakra is divided into areas of the clock that have previously been described. Figure 4.2 shows this. The region around 12 o'clock is related to our spiritual self and also to karma. This region I call **HEAVEN**. The whole of the middle, that I call **EARTH** is related to the physical body and all the incumbent internal organs and systems. The lower region at around 6 o'clock is related to our ancestry (sometimes called miasm), called **MAN**. The 3 o'clock region tells us if the dis-ease emanates from emotional causes and the 9 o'clock region tells us if dis-ease emanates from the physical causes. The illustration also shows how the Crown chakra is related to our spirituality, the Base chakra to our ancestry and familial tendencies whilst the Heart chakra is in the very centre of our being (as it is in our physical body).

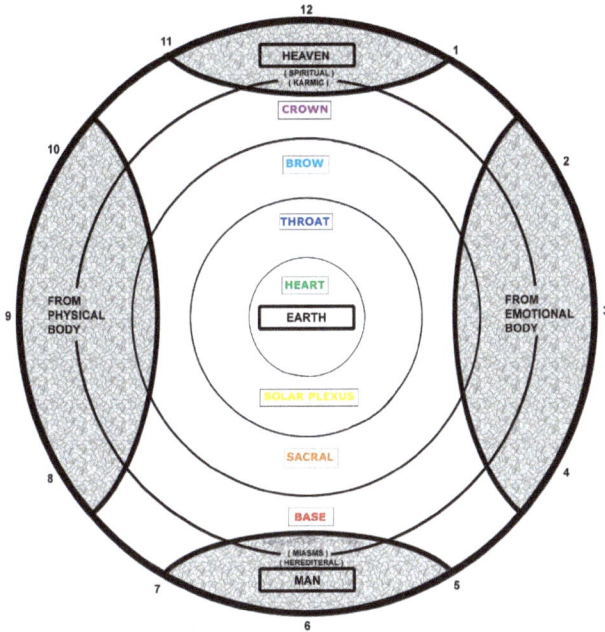

Figure 4.2

Interpretation of a Major Chakra at the Etheric/Emotional Level

So when we detect an energy imbalance at 12 o'clock, it signifies that it is due to our karma and there is very little that can be done to alter symptoms with any form of healing. When energy imbalance is detected around the 6 o'clock region it signifies that it is an herediteral condition and one of predisposition. Whether or not one is able to alter this situation depends on your philosophy. I personally believe that it *is* possible to ease symptoms that are congenital and herediteral with specific constitutional homoeopathy. Certain very gifted healers are also capable of treating these symptoms, but I don't believe it can be achieved with distance healing. When you become experienced at feeling above the Witness at the Emotional Body level, you will be able to detect imbalance within the 'body' of the chakra that relates to the levels between the Crown and Base. For instance, if you feel an energy imbalance (fizzing) at the very centre of the circle, that will indicate an imbalance in the Heart chakra at that level. It is, however, the 3 o'clock and 9 o'clock regions that are the most important as to proffering advice to your client. Energy imbalance at the 3 o'clock region signifies that this imbalance is from our emotions and imbalance at 9 o'clock signifies that it heralds from the abusing of our body, such as incorrect diet or excesses in many other fields. Healing at these two sites should be accompanied with communication to the client regarding the cause.

THE MENTAL BODY

Overview

The final subtle body that we may utilise in distance healing is the Mental Body. It is said to be the lowest of the 'higher' or spiritual self. It can extend as much as 75 cms (30 inches) away from the physical body and it is obvious it is much subtler than anything that have been previously mentioned. For distance healing above the Witness, you can affect the Mental Body at around 30 cms (12 inches). The substance that makes up the Mental Body concerns thoughts and mental processes called 'thought forms'. In simple language, when we think, this is the region where or thoughts originate. If we show love and positivity, this will affect our endocrine system and autonomic nervous system that alters our blood chemistry, hormonal levels and organic secretions. Negative thought will eventually destroy us. We are totally responsible for our own health, or as much of our health as we have been granted at conception and birth, bearing in mind that various environmental factors also affect us. Many of our psychosomatic and mental imbalance stems from imbalance within the Mental Body. Some authorities would say that the Mental Body is responsible for our character and personality. I disagree, in that I believe that these are initiated from many different sources.

Healing

Following the initial work on the Witness as previously described, take the dominant or both hands to a height at least 30 cms (12 inches) above the witness. Then proceed to scan a large circle, about the size of a large dinner plate or at least 12 inches in diameter, very slowly and purposefully. You must keep your eyes and focus riveted on the **MENTAL** box at all times. When you find an area of energy imbalance or hot spot, there will be some altered sensation – see below for details. With Mental Body healing there is no need to energy balance with the coupled chakra. All that is required is that you accept the imbalance that is being given to you and dwell very still on that area whilst saying similar words or incantations as previously described. If you are working at this high level you are usually asking for healing to be sent to the *whole person*, not to any particular chakra, internal organ or system. What I generally do is to ask for healing of the whole person via the Crown chakra and ask that healing pervades their whole being. Therefore, it helps to have an image of the client in front of you, a photograph as well as the witness is a good idea or simply just to write down their name will suffice.

Sensations under the fingers

Once again there may be a myriad of sensations ranging from fizzing, buzzing, electric shock sensation. Increased warmth doesn't usually occur and certainly not any degree of buffering or a barrier sensation. The healing has been successful when the sensation ceases. This is often accompanied with you taking a deep breath or having a tingling sensation. On the whole, the sensations you feel at this level are much lighter than the Emotional Body.

Summary of the conditions and symptoms with each subtle body in healing mode

Physical Body

You will send healing to the Physical Body for any injuries and accidents that have been caused by external trauma. These will include musculo-skeletal conditions including repetitive strains and cuts and bruises. Don't be tempted to send healing through the Physical Body to such conditions as osteo-arthritis or any musculo-skeletal conditions that were not caused by trauma.

Etheric Body

You will send healing to the client through their Etheric Body for the following: - Osteo-arthritis; Spinal arthritis; Spinal conditions; Endocrine imbalance; Hormonal imbalance; Oedema; Lymphatic and Circulatory conditions but not internal Heart conditions; Headaches/Migraine if caused by mechanical or cerebro-spinal fluid flow imbalance; Throat, Ear and Eye conditions in general; Menopausal and Menstrual imbalance; acute Stomach and Bowel upset; This Body covers everything associated with fluid flow symptoms that have not been caused by emotional upsets.

Emotional Body

 As stated earlier in the book, most of our chronic conditions become symptomatic in the body due to Emotional Body energy imbalance. So as well as the obvious emotions such as tearfulness, anxiety, grief etc. Emotional Body healing will also cover all internal organic conditions such as all chronic (long standing) conditions of the Ear, Nose and Throat; Respiratory; Abdominal and Bowel; Genito-Urinary; Heart; Liver; Dermatological and some Neurological conditions to include Sleep disorders; Headaches; Migraine; Hypertension; Tinnitus; Overweight tendencies et al.

Mental Body

You may send healing through the Mental Body to treat anything previously mentioned if it is arrowed to the Crown chakra. Generally, though you would use the Mental Body to send healing for Mental imbalance such as Depression, Chronic Anxiety, Insecurity; Phobias and Fears; Low Self Esteem and Introvertness

The above list is not exhaustive and there are several overlaps with some conditions. If you are unsure which subtle body to use for your healing – just ask!

CONCLUSION

It is my earnest wish that this short book will be of help to anyone who wishes to use this wonderful form of healing but is unsure as to the 'nuts and bolts' of it. It has been a delight to be able to share my knowledge with you all. I am always available to answer any queries you may have by sending me an email to jrcacupressure@hotmail.com Details of my other books and A1 clinical posters are available from www.johncrosspublications.com

Dr John R Cross FCSP

12 Upper Milovaig

Glendale

Isle of Skye

IV55 8WY, Scotland

April 2016

BIBLIOGRAPHY

Bloy, C. *I'm Just Going Down to the Pub to Do a Few Miracles.* Devon, England: Fountain International, 1990

Brennan, B.A. *Hands of Light: A Guide to Healing Through the Human Energy Field*. New York: Bantam, 1987

Cross, J.R. *Healing with the Chakra Energy System. Acupressure, Bodywork and Reflexology for Total Health.* Berkeley, Calif. North Atlantic Books, 2006

Cross, J.R. *Acupuncture and the Chakra Energy System – Treating the Cause of Disease.* Berkeley, Calif. North Atlantic Books, 2008

Dale, C. *The Subtle Body – An Encyclopaedia of Your Energetic Anatomy.* Boulder, Colorado. Sounds True, 2009

Motoyama, H. *Theories of the Chakras: Bridge to Higher Consciousness*. Theosophical Publishing House, 1988

Smith, C.W. *Electromagnetics and the Autonomic Nervous System*. Based upon lecture given at the 25th annual symposium to On Man and His Environment in Health and Disease given on June 7th 2007

Tansley, D.V. *Radionics and the Subtle Anatomy of Man*. Cambridge, England. C.W. Daniel 1972

www.ingramcontent.com/pod-product-compliance
Lightning Source LLC
Chambersburg PA
CBHW041224270326
41933CB00001B/44